BACK PAIN
... were turned on...
the last *don't panic!* ...

Cover illustration reproduced with kind permission of Ralph Steadman

# BACK PAIN

*don't panic!*

Peter G Skew
MBBS, LRCP, MRCS, DipM-SMed
*Vice President*
*British Institute of Musculoskeletal Medicine*
*34 Park Avenue*
*Watford, UK*

**MARTIN DUNITZ**

© Martin Dunitz Ltd 2000

First published in the United Kingdom in 2000 by
Martin Dunitz Ltd
The Livery House
7–9 Pratt Street
London NW1 0AE

Tel: +44 (0)20 7482 2202
Fax: +44 (0)20 7267 0159

A CIP catalogue record for this book is available from the British
Library.

ISBN 1-85317-957-4

Composition by Scribe Design, Gillingham, Kent
Printed and bound in Italy by Printer Trento S.r.l.

# *Contents*

This book was written to help doctors treat patients and patients to help themselves. It came about for a number of reasons. Firstly, I really enjoy treating back pain and find it deeply rewarding; secondly, many patients suffer unnecessarily for many years with treatable conditions; thirdly, I feel sympathetic towards my colleagues who do not find treating back pain enjoyable ...

Back pain is an almost universal heart sink condition for doctors and sufferers alike and has been used as a social excuse by patients suffering from depression or unhappiness at work. In the 1990s the British government colluded with this by making it more financially attractive to be on invalidity benefit rather than unemployment benefit. For generations, doctors' education regarding this common condition has been non-existent; combine this with a lack of research in this area, and it is no wonder that few doctors 'care' for this condition.

My strongest memory of my general practitioner attachment, as a student, at the age of 20 is of a large builder, in serious pain with backache, who had to be helped to climb the stairs to a grand consulting room in Bath by his 5-year-old daughter. After what I now know to be a cursory examination and an unrefined manipulation, this man scooped up his daughter in one arm and trotted down the stairs free of pain. For me this was what being a doctor meant, direct doctor input leading to patient recovery.

Several years of indoctrination and house jobs later, I managed to learn these techniques, and others, from my GP trainers, from private specialist manipulators and on courses run by the British Association of Manipulative Medicine.

I find the stimulation and challenge of dealing with back pain is always fresh, as few patients have the same mix of premorbid personality, injury, social circumstances or reaction to pain. This view of the challenge is what I wish to share with my colleagues.

Recent publications on evidence and reviews by the Clinical Standards Advisory Group on Back Pain 1994 prompted guidelines published by the Royal College of General Practitioners 1996, relaunched with revisions 1999 (see *Appendix 1*). These excellent outlines have provided the bones of understanding; I wish to put some philosophical muscle on them to allow back pain to come alive.

GPs cannot be fully aware of all aspects of medicine—for me, nephrology, lipid metabolism, diabetes and ophthalmology have all been subjects to avoid. However, even with avoided subjects, it is necessary to have enough knowledge to know when to refer a patient and to have an appropriate referral pathway. As regards back pain, and indeed all musculoskeletal disorders, teaching is absent in medical schools and only available as a postgraduate topic if sought out. At present, an appropriate referral pathway does not exist, which leaves most GPs with little knowledge and no backup.

Apprehension + ignorance + pain = panic

*but*

reassurance + education + pain relief ... result ... no panic

## *The size of the problem*

Back pain is an enormous problem. This statement will have few dissenters, but what does this mean to us individually, to society, employers, insurers and the government—especially the departments of Health (DoH), Social Security (DSS), Trade (DoT) and Environment, Transport and the Regions (DETR)?

In all, 60–80% of individuals will experience back pain at some time in their life. The Health and Safety Executive (HSE) estimates that there are more than half a million people suffering from work-related back pain at any one time. DETR figures show musculoskeletal problems to be the cause of 50% of work absences, of which back pain represents more than half. The cost to industry is about £5 billion, the cost to the NHS is £481 million, with over 12 million GP consultations. Yet most doctors have next to no preparation or teaching on this subject at any time in either under- or post-graduate medical training. Thus it is not surprising that a recent trial conducted at several practices prospectively over 1 year showed that after 3 months patients stopped going to see their GP, but at 12 months 75% still had back pain symptoms which were significant to them (Croft et al, 1998).

In society as a whole many people are not involving themselves in various activities owing to back pain; every year, football and other team sports lose participants as a result of back pain. Playing with the children or standing to have a drink in the pub become difficult and more pain than pleasure. Lifting the baby from the cot is no longer fun but a painful chore.

In 1995, back pain cost employers about 5.5 million days in lost production, plus sick pay, retraining, recruitment costs, loss of skills and increased insurance premiums. Insurers pay out millions through permanent health insurance and employers' liability claims for back pain, and self-insuring employers such as the Fire Service and the Police have to take funds from services to pay for ill health retirement, in many instances for back pain. Government costs are many, and are easily dismissed; however, the only money that the government has to spend comes from all of us in taxes, so we should care.

The National Health Service (NHS), as will be discussed, fails to provide an appropriate service. Although back pain is relatively easy to treat in the acute phase, waiting lists guarantee that this opportunity is missed. This leaves the NHS treating chronic pain, which is widely recognized as a different and more difficult problem. At this point the costs of repeated consultations at GP and specialist level are high, as costs of high-tech investigations and pain clinic sessions are much higher than appropriate early interventions (J Campbell, 1998, personal communication).

The Department of Social Security, like private insurers, pays out huge sums for sickness and invalidity benefit, figures which have risen exponentially in recent years. Local government is a major employer and it loses resources directly in the same way as other employers from the effects of back pain.

## History and epidemiology

Early books carry pictures of equipment and techniques for traction and treatment of back pain, confirming the long-standing nature of the problem. However, it is almost unknown in so-called primitive cultures, some of which do not even have a word for the complaint. A search of *MedLine* revealed that the highest rates of back pain are in the high income countries such as Sweden, Germany and Belgium. In low income countries rates of back pain were higher in urban than in rural populations and still higher amongst workers in enclosed workshops. In European countries alone hard physical labour was not directly correlated with incidence of back pain. High rates in low income populations in enclosed workshops and low incidence in low income farmers suggests a social influence as an aetiological factor.

## Human design

Is back pain genetic? Is it due to a design fault? Recent twin studies at St Thomas's Hospital (London) showed that 60% of spinal degeneration is genetic, but this does not equate with back pain (Sambrook, 1999). Some conditions, such as spondylolisthesis, appear to be congenital; 25% of cases occur in families. Scoliosis appears to be congenital, and like spina bifida of minor degrees, it is often asymptomatic, only being found at investigation for some other condition. There are few conditions that predictably lead to back pain.

So often, even from well educated doctors interested in back pain, the argument is put forward that as bipeds we are hampered by a spine designed for quadrupeds. We have been bipedal for in excess of 2 million years, during which time we have undergone significant development and evolution; it would be a real surprise if something as basic as the spine had not developed satisfactorily. Creationists would say we were designed to be upright and Darwinists must accept the argument that enough time has passed to allow for evolution to have worked. So what is the problem?

We rely on our spines to hold us up, but our skeletons are not designed to do this unaided. In the 1980s Professor Punjabi of the Yale University School of Medicine carried out an experiment whereby, after removing all the muscles from a healthy spine, he subjected it to increasing weight while maintaining it in a neutral position. After only 2 kg, which is about one-fifth the weight of the head, the spine buckled and became unstable. Like a tent, the spine needs guy ropes (muscles) for support at rest and during movement; it also needs muscles to produce the movement. These roles are performed by different types of muscle, primary stabilizers, which are short muscles between adjacent vertebrae, and primary movers, which are longer muscles with more leverage, running over several segments, to superficial muscles which run from the base of the skull to the sacrum. This is in fact a wonderful piece of design. So, again, what is the problem?

As probably the most complex organism on the planet with the most chromosomes we humans should expect to be the slowest to evolve genetically to changes in our environment. However, we have changed our environment more quickly in the last 50 years than at any time in our evolutionary history.

My answer to the question is that we have stopped using ourselves as we have evolved to function.

**Table 1**
*Comparison of activities, AD 1–2000*

| Parameter | Year 1 | Year 2000 | Effect on back pain |
|-----------|--------|-----------|---------------------|
| Walking | More | Less | Negative |
| Sitting | Less | More | Negative |
| Driving | None | More | Negative |
| Manual work | More | Less | Neutral |
| Obesity | Less | More | Negative |
| Smoking | Less | More | Negative |
| Age (life expectancy) | <40 | >70 | Negative |

If we take a conservative estimate that it takes a hundred generations for humans to adapt to a change in the environment, with a generation being about 20 years, that means we are genetically adapted to life as lived at the time of Christ. We will therefore only be adapted to our current lifestyle in 2000 years time. This does not help us today. However, if we look at the differences between today's lifestyle and that of 2000 years ago we may identify some of the triggers of back pain (Table 1).

If we did less of what modern man does and more of what 1st century man did, we would be using our spine as it evolved to be used. After all, you would not buy a Rolls Royce to plough fields.

## Causes of back pain

Most sufferers want to know what is causing their pain: a diagnosis is required. In the case of back pain, it is often difficult to provide such a diagnosis. However, if the patient acquires some knowledge about what might cause the pain, far less anxiety may be generated.

### Tissues with pain sensors

To make some sense of the causes of back pain, let us look at the tissues of the back and take both a structural and functional view of pain. To produce a pain sensation, tissues need nociceptors or pain sensors (Figure 1; for more details see the chapter on *Acute pain, chronic pain and the transition between them*). These are present in periosteum, the outer third of the annulus fibrosus (the fibrous part of the intervertebral disc) and in ligaments of the spine (intervertebral and ligamentum flavum). The joint capsules of the zygoapophyseal joints have nociceptors, as have the muscles and fascia between them. These receptors are designed to respond to local stimuli, tissue damage, release of inflammatory mediators, cytokines and other substances and excess stress or pressure, as a protective function to stop further damage.

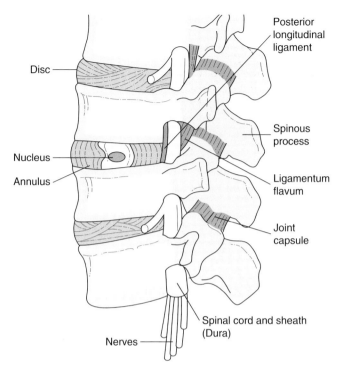

**Figure 1**
*Tissues with pain sensors.*

One mechanism that acts to stop the further damage is muscle spasm, which restricts the movement that aggravates pain. Spasm in turn leads to ischaemia owing to restricted blood and tissue fluid circulation and the generation of muscle or myofascial trigger points, another painful condition. Nerve sheaths and dura are rich in nociceptors and can produce pains which are difficult to localize, as both segmental and referred pain patterns occur. Stimulation of any of these tissues will lead to a pain sensation being recorded in the brain, with varying degrees of accuracy for localization.

# *Mechanisms of pain sensor stimulation*

## Pressure

This is the most important mechanism of nociceptor stimulation in mechanical back pain (Figure 2). Pressure within the disc causes no pain until any fractures of the annulus reach the outer third. The resulting disc pain is aggravated by movements which change the pressure on the nociceptors. Pressure or stretching of ligaments by bulging discs secondary to loss of disc height or prolapse of the nucleus also stimulates receptors. Direct pressure on nerve sheaths and nerves leads to the classic distribution of sciatica if the pressure is on the L5, S1,2 roots.

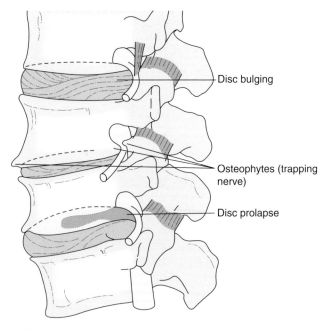

Disc bulging

Osteophytes (trapping nerve)

Disc prolapse

**Figure 2**
*Pressure points around the spinal joints.*

Pressure on the sheath alone gives pain. Pressure on the whole nerve leads to pain, numbness and weakness in the distribution of the nerve root. These pressure stimuli can come from discs bulging or prolapsing, thickened ligaments or osteophytes around joints.

Pressure is also the stimulus for facet joint pain and ligament pain (Figure 3). As a result of disc deterioration and general wear the facet joints take an increasing proportion of the weight of the upper body. This increase in pressure and wear over time leads to degeneration, osteoarthrosis and osteophyte formation. The small inclusion bodies/miniscoids and fat pads within the facet joint under this increased pressure may be compressed, damaged or extruded from the joint into the recesses of the joint capsule. This and effusions in the joints put pressure on the richly innervated ligaments of the capsule, causing some of the pain of facet joint dysfunction.

Pressure arising from tension in muscles is one mechanism for pain coming directly from muscles in spasm.

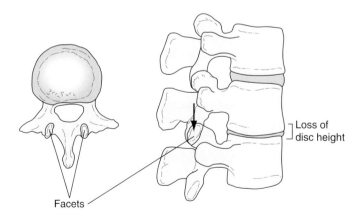

Loss of disc height

Facets

*Figure 3*
*Transfer of pressure to zygoapophyseal joints (facet joints) with disc degeneration: the three joint complex.*

Tension transferred to the attachment of the muscle tendon to the bone creates micro-injury/trauma, creating a situation similar to that found in tennis elbow, but situated deep to the back muscles close to the spine where localization of the pain is very difficult. In this situation recurrent injury adds up to chronic pain.

## Chemical irritation

Chemical irritation of nociceptors is the other major pain stimulus, and follows tissue trauma with localized bleeding. Cell damage releases inflammatory mediators, which attract repair cells from the blood and surrounding tissues. As regards back pain, these causes of pain are short-lived, the repair process taking 7–10 days, as with other injuries. The local response of the muscles is a secondary effect of spasm leading to dysfunction of neighbouring joints, which takes the mechanism back to pressure of one kind or another. The mechanism changes with time from chemical to mechanical, from injury to dysfunction, which then affects adjacent areas of the spine and the area affected grows.

## *Dysfunctional causes of back pain*

Back pain symptoms are often of sudden onset, but are in fact the result of long-standing changes to the skeleton, muscular system and posture which have finally reached the stage where the body can no longer compensate. The body has an in-built ability to compensate called homoeostasis. Compare the tolerance of the other systems of the body: 60% of liver function must be lost before symptoms occur, one kidney or one lung may be lost and adequate function retained, only 40% of coronary artery function remains at the onset of angina symptoms. It is not really surprising that 'acute' back pain takes so long to settle, the symptoms are recent (i.e. acute), but the cause or causes may well have been developing for many years and represent long-standing weakness of muscles, dysfunction of joints and general neglect. The situation can be likened to the way that a string rubbing or chaffing on a rough edge for a long time 'suddenly' lets go. These factors develop slowly, compromising the functional co-ordination of the structures of the spine necessary for support and movement.

Movement is the key function of the spine which is often overlooked. Stability and flexibility are inevitable results of the structure of the spine. Compare the shoulder joint which is like 'a ball on a plate', highly mobile but unstable, with the hip joint which exhibits excellent stability but limited movement. Considering the forces which run through it the spine is very flexible, notably in two areas, the cervical (neck region) and the lower back (lumbar region), where the ribs do not have a splinting effect. A disproportionate amount of symptoms arise in these two regions—especially the adjacent junctions, occipitocervical, cervicothoracic, thoracolumbar and lumbosacral.

The bones are joined by ligaments which form the capsule of the facet joints and pass around the disc. As in most joints, the ligaments are protected by the muscles, which also move the joints. In the spine, adjacent bones are moved on each other by short muscles called the rotatores, intertransversarii and multifidus. These muscles cause rotation and side bending, but they are primarily stabilizers in this function, not movers; the movers are longer muscles, especially the oblique muscles of the abdominal wall for rotation, quadratus lumborum for side bending and erector spinae for extension. This in some way explains why back pain accompanies activities like hoovering and ironing, especially after childbirth or an abdominal operation, which weaken abdominal muscles. Having lost the function of weakened prime movers, the short muscles are used inappropriately and become strained.

The functional relationship between joints and muscles is generally understood and accepted, as is the innervation. Movement in the spine is initiated by powerful muscles which run over several spinal segments, making the relationships more complex than with other joints. Coordination failure, i.e. dysfunction or injury, of any muscle will influence the joints over which it runs and vice versa (Figure 4). This explains how symptoms may manifest themselves well away from the immediate site of injury, current or previous, and still be linked causally. Individual small injuries or dysfunctions summate over time and cause other muscular or postural changes to occur, leading to incoordination of movement and predisposing to more problems. In this insidious way simple things

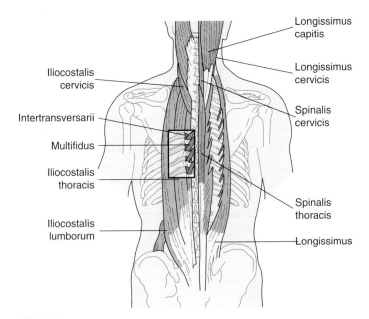

*Figure 4*
*Muscles of the back: the short muscles are stabilisers, and the long muscles are movers.*

become complex. This is all happening all the time to everyone's backs; with exercise and significant movement a lot is naturally corrected at this structural level. The problem is that the body is connected to a mind, and in back pain more than most other conditions, mental state is a stronger predictor of outcome than other factors.

As will be seen in the subsequent chapters, movement is the key feature of treatment of most spinal disorders.

## *Sources of confusion*

Our understanding of physiological pain is that it prevents further damage by stopping further movements. Paradoxically, this understanding impedes progress in treating back pain and many other musculoskeletal disorders.

Facet joint dysfunction and muscle spasm both cause pain, but neither is associated with actual or potential tissue damage, so pain should not impede movement. In both these situations movement is the treatment required to restore function.

In chronic micro-trauma of the spinal ligaments, the treatment should be the same as for tennis elbow: injection of local anaesthetic and steroid, deep friction massage and stretching—a movement which causes pain but not further damage.

With torn muscles, in the thigh for instance, after sufficient time for healing the next phase of treatment is stretching, which is painful but strongly acknowledged to be essential for adequate treatment.

Why should we not treat the back in exactly the same way, and accept that some treatments are painful but necessary? The answer is that back pain comes fully equipped with its own type of panic that abolishes rational thought. The lack of satisfactory research and consensus on how to treat back pain also allows doubt and confusion to have access to the process for doctor and patient alike.

## *Symptoms and signs produced by various tissues*

The tissues being stimulated determine where the pain is felt, but these links are not always straightforward. Having described the tissues which may cause pain and how they may be stimulated, it is important to point out the symptoms and signs that each tissue may produce. More than one problem may be present, i.e. disc degeneration, bulging discs pressing on ligaments, osteophytes and joint dysfunction can all occur together; but one or more factors may cause symptoms at any one time.

### Bones

Infection and malignancy lead to local tenderness and constant pain—especially at night—which is often unchanged by movement. They may also cause general symptoms such as weight loss, temperature and fatigue. Fracture gives local tenderness, constant pain and pain on movement following a history of trauma. The trauma may be very slight in some susceptible groups, particularly in Asians, AIDS patients, smokers, elderly women, those with a history of steroid use or other risk factors for osteoporosis and people with scoliosis.

### Discs

Degeneration causes central pain that is dull in nature, worse after bending forwards and aggravated by movement to extremes in all directions. Disc fractures and partial disc prolapses are characterized by pain on some movements but not others, i.e. pain on right side bending and extension but not left side bending, flexion or rotation to either side. A characteristic tilt may also be present, caused by 'protective' muscle spasm. Complete disc prolapse causes symptoms related to the tissues it presses on.

## Joints

The cartilage, inclusion bodies, capsule and ligaments of the joints are innervated by the nerves that run past the joint. These nerves supply the associated segment, and symptoms from joint problems are often felt around the segment as referred pain (see Figure 6). Pain is unilateral, aggravated by some movements which produce common pressure upon the joint, e.g. flexion, left side bending and rotation to the right produce common tensile pressure on the right facet joint. Similarly, extension, left side bending and rotation to the right produce common compressive pressure on the left facet joint. Both the above examples produce pain on the same movements but the pain is on the side of the lesion, i.e. right in the first example and left in the second. History in these cases may well be of an awkward movement or sitting awkwardly rather than heavy lifting or injury. The sacro-iliac joint is somewhat different from other joints, being mostly fibrous. Disruption at this joint occurs by jarring through the leg missing a step or sitting down hard on one side; symptoms are low back pain, local tenderness over the joint or referred pain into the groin. Symptoms are aggravated by stressing the joint.

## Ligaments

The ligamentum flavum is richly innervated and produces symptoms of a central distribution when stretched. Other ligaments give symptoms in characteristic areas, identified in the 1950s, with little regard for segmental neurology or

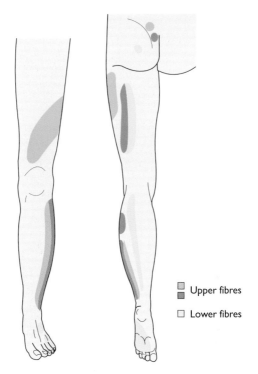

**Figure 5**
*Referred pain in non-segmental pattern from posterior sacroiliac ligament strain. (Adapted from Hackett GS, Ligament and Tendon Relaxation Treated by Prolotherapy, 3rd edn, 1958. Courtesy of Charles C Thomas, Publisher, Ltd, Springfield, Illinois.)*

Upper fibres

Lower fibres

conventional referral patterns (Figure 5). The history would be of extreme flexion, side bending or extension; pain on movement is at the end range when the ligament is under tension. Sprained, strained or loose ligaments are implicated by many authorities as the most common cause of chronic back pain. If this is so, despite the severity and longevity of the pain a sprained ligament should not be a source of anxiety. Just understanding the mechanism should reassure the sufferer and hence reduce the perceived pain.

## Nerves

Irritation of nerve sheaths creates pain in the distribution of the nerve, i.e. segmental, and is aggravated by nerve stretching, but pins and needles, numbness or weakness are absent. More severe compression of the nerve leads to pins and needles, numbness and weakness, as well as pain in the root distribution (Figure 6).

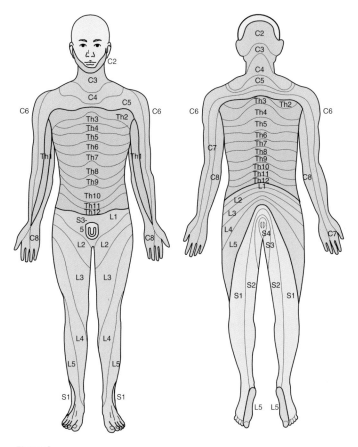

**Figure 6**
*Nerve root distribution.*

***Table 2***
*Root links to muscles and reflexes.*

| Nerve origin | Muscle | Function |
|---|---|---|
| C1 | Sternomastoid | Rotation of neck |
| C2, 3, 4 | Trapezius | Shrugging of shoulders |
| C5 | Deltoid and supraspinatus | Abduction of shoulder |
| C5 | Infraspinatus | External rotation of shoulder |
| C5, 6 | Biceps brachii | Flexion of elbow |
| C6 | Extensor carpi | Extension of wrist |
| C7 | Latissimus dorsi | Arm adduction |
| C7 | Common flexors | Wrist flexion |
| C7 | Triceps | Extension of elbow |
| C8 | Flexor and extensor carpi ulnaris | Ulnar deviation of wrist |
| C8 | Extensor pollicis | Extension of thumb |
| C8 | Adductor pollicis | Adduction of thumb |
| C8 | Extensor digitorum | Extension of fingers |
| T1 | Interossei | Approximation ring and little finger |
| L2, 3 | Psoas | Hip flexion |
| L3 | Quadriceps femoris | Knee extension |
| L4 | Tibialis anterior | Dorsiflexion of ankle |
| L4, 5 | Extensor hallucis | Great toe extension |
| L5 | Gluteus medius | Hip abduction |
| L5, S1 | Peronei | Eversion of foot |
| S1, 2 | Gastrocnemius/soleus | Plantar flexion of foot |
| S1, 2 | Hamstrings | Knee flexion |
| S1, 2 | | Gluteal wasting |

**Reflexes**

| | | |
|---|---|---|
| C5, 6 | Biceps | |
| C5, 6 | Supinator | |
| C7 | Triceps | |
| L3 | Quadriceps | |
| S1 | Ankle jerk | |

Table 2 outlines root links to muscle weakness and reflex changes. Pain may be electrical in nature, like banging the funny bone, and this is aggravated on stretching by straight leg raising in the lower limb or various neural tension tests for the upper limb.

## Muscles

Tears, sprains and strains of muscles in the back occur with unaccustomed exercise, over-use or direct injury; local pain and tenderness are major symptoms. Pain is aggravated by stretching the muscle passively, using the muscle actively and especially by resisted testing (see Cyriax's publications; *Appendix 2*).

## Fascia

Symptoms generated in fascia are often referred away from the site of origin of the problem, which may be a trigger point. Excellent examples are given in works by Travell and Simons (see *Appendix 2*). The major characteristic is that the pain referral is not segmental (see *Related conditions*).

## Skin

It is often forgotten that skin can be the site of a problem giving back pain. Early shingles may present with unilateral pain and skin sensitivity before other signs or symptoms, and other forms of radiculitis are also possible.

## Internal organs

Back pain from internal organs is dealt with in the chapter on *Related conditions* as non-back causes of back pain.

## Grades of back pain

Severity of pain may conveniently be measured by the visual analogue scale (VAS; Figure 7), which is a 10 cm

Patient's side of scale

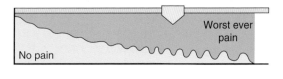

Doctor's side of scale

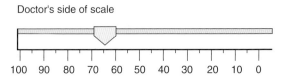

**Figure 7**
*Visual analogue scale.*

scale marked from 0 to 100 representing no pain to excruciating pain. The use of this scheme for assessing back pain gives three broad categories of this condition that directly correlate with levels of anxiety.

Mild back pain with a VAS value between 10 and 30 following unaccustomed exercise, with a readily identifiable cause, is not associated with anxiety, e.g. following a weekend's gardening. Healing takes place after 6 or 7 days, during which time function is not lost, as pain is only minimal or easily controlled by simple pain relief. This condition is almost an old friend of gardeners and DIY enthusiasts, occurring with changing activities. A potential for episodes of aggravation exists with the muscular stiffness of unaccustomed exercise if further awkward movements are undertaken. With an understandable cause, continued activity and spontaneous resolution or resolution following prompt appropriate treatment, e.g. osteopathic or chiropractic, there is no panic.

Moderate pain (30–60 on the scale) is more significant, not controlled immediately with analgesics. Sleep is disturbed and doubt creeps in. This level of pain perceived in a first episode, accompanied by severe muscle spasm, may engender more anxiety and apprehension. When the problem has been created by an awkward movement, an obvious cause may not be discernible, the pain may continue to increase relatively slowly over 3 or 4 days, reducing mobility and encouraging rest as a treatment rather than a necessity. Movement-generated pain may come in severe spasms, causing involuntary gasps. Sleep disturbance is considerable, stiffness getting out of bed in the morning is significant. Pain may well be improved only by the addition of alcohol or heat to the pain killer ... panic appears.

Severe pain (>60 on the scale) is more likely to follow an accident or trauma of some kind—a fall or a work or sporting injury. Early investigation by X-ray is essential to exclude a displaced fracture, which may need fixation, or other fractures needing rest and support only, and follow-up to confirm healing. With any type of fracture great care must be taken to avoid lifting until healing has occurred. With all ligament or muscle tears and fractures pain is aggravated by specific movements and restricted by muscle spasm. Response to pain relief, heat and rest is less complete, fear, apprehension, anxiety levels are high ... panic is established at an early stage.

This is a good time to move on to the subject of treatment.

## Treatment

All treatments are applied on the background of natural healing, so some knowledge of that process is essential so that any treatment given can be assessed accurately.

## Natural healing

All tissues, with the exception of nerves, heal by fibrosis, regeneration and remodelling, leaving various degrees of scarring. Nerves comprise cell projections (axons) running in 'conduits' (nerve sheaths). Provided that the 'conduit' is unbroken, the nerve cell can regrow slowly (about one inch per month) to reconnect following damage. If the nerve sheath is severed reconnection is not possible unless the nerve is sewn together and then reconnection is a matter of luck.

Bone heals well; it is remodelled over time, obeying Woolf's 'law of bone transformation' published in 1892, which stated simply that 'form follows function'. Only slight thickness remains to demonstrate the history. Bone is a structural element which continues as before the injury.

Muscle heals fairly well, with fibrosis, no remodelling and some scarring, which is a little weaker than the original tissue. Muscle is a functional tissue, scar is inert, so restoration of function in muscle relies on development of undamaged fibres by exercise after healing has taken place.

Ligaments heal by fibrosis and scarring, which is very similar to the original structure, and the orientation of the scar is significantly improved by passive stretching and active movement. Ligament is inactive tissue and scarring sometimes leads to strengthening; this is used as a treatment in sclerosant therapy. However, ligaments may become lax with repeated injury, leading to an abnormal degree of joint movement, regarded by some as the commonest cause of chronic back pain.

Joint capsules tear, cartilage surfaces over bone can crack and bruise, and inclusion bodies in the joint may be damaged, but little is known of the specific results of healing in this area, which will be by scarring and may reduce joint mobility. Recurrent micro-trauma and scarring may be a cause of chronic back pain, as this area is well innervated.

Discs have a very limited blood supply, degenerate with repeated trauma, dehydrate and undergo fibrous replacement. Prolapsed discs often naturally reduce in size over 6–12 months.

*Healing times* vary greatly, depending on the site and size of injury. Specifically, in the spine bones heal in 6–12 weeks, ligaments and micro-fractures at the enthesis take 4–8 weeks and muscles take 2–4 weeks to heal. However, it takes another 4 weeks or so to achieve full strength in the scar and several more weeks of exercise to re-establish the original strength of the muscle. Satisfactory healing of all tissues can be expected within about 8 weeks, so rehabilitation even from quite severe injury can start by then. Ideally, rehabilitation of non-painful areas should start earlier.

# General principles and strategies of treatment

The preceding chapters have been designed to show a complex layered structure with complex inter-relationships between structures and between structure and function. Overlap of symptoms and signs occurs; therefore only detailed history, examination and investigation by a well trained and experienced doctor can possibly result in the establishment of even a tentative diagnosis. True. Except that, other than so-called red flag disorders—i.e. possible serious spinal pathology including infection, fracture, cancer, osteoporosis or spinal tumour—and the not so red flag conditions such as nerve root pain caused by compression, all other conditions are simply treated the same. Thus the term simple back pain can be applied, because the treatment is simple. An accurate diagnosis is rarely necessary unless simple treatments fail to ease the problem within 4 weeks.

---

The simple treatment is:

- pain relief
- maintenance of function
- increase range of movement
- increase strength
- increase stability and coordination
- prevention of recurrence (often omitted).

---

These are the cornerstones of treatment for back pain whatever the cause and whichever treatment modality is used.

## Treatment options

*General treatments* common to several treatment modalities include heat and/or ice to reduce pain, stimulate blood flow and the healing process by clearing bruising and bringing the appropriate blood cells (macrophages) to clear up the damaged tissue. Massage also improves blood flow, reduces swelling and improves function. Exercises are used for mobility and strengthening to prevent recurrence.

*Acupuncture* is available in several guises of varying value in the treatment of back pain. Classical Chinese acupuncture comprises a whole system of diagnosis and treatment developed over 2000 ago and uses different parameters to those used and understood by Western doctors and patients. For some conditions associated with back pain, which have general causes or are related to internal organ dysfunction leading to symptoms clustered on one side of the body, Chinese acupuncture may be the only system by which all the symptoms may be linked. More useful for European patients is the system of acupuncture developed and taught by Felix Mann; details are given in *Appendix 2*. A third form of acupuncture has been proposed by Chan Gunn, called 'intramuscular stimulation'. This technique is well described in his book (see *Appendix 2*); the basis of this treatment is needling muscles that are acutely or chronically in spasm. This technique may reverse spasm in deep muscles which has been present for years, causing persistent widespread and intractable symptoms. Its use in well chosen cases can have startling effects with regard to pain relief and improvement in mobility. If the technique is followed by a full rehabilitation programme to restore strength it is possible to achieve astonishing results.

*Allopathic treatments* are those provided through the NHS, by the GP in most cases, and can be broken down into those aimed at the healing process, pain relief and prevention of recurrence.

Physiotherapy offers various approaches to the treatment of back pain. These include ultrasound, which reduces swelling and increases blood flow, and interferential therapy, an electrical treatment which stimulates the muscles by encouraging gentle contractions and also increases blood supply to the area, thus promoting healing and encouraging stronger healing. Laser treatment is a newer modality that uses laser light to stimulate tissues to a depth of 1–2 cm; this seems to have a very positive effect on scar formation, resulting in smaller firmer scars. Ultrasound and interferential treatments are effective for back conditions where laser therapy does not penetrate deeply enough to be of much use, but may help following surgery to improve scar quality.

Drugs can help shorten the healing process directly by reducing further damage caused by the healing process. Following tissue damage bruising occurs as a result of blood entering the tissues; this causes the release of inflammatory mediators, including cytokinins; these attract blood cells which destroy damaged tissue. Sometimes these cells destroy more tissue than is necessary, and anti-inflammatory drugs can moderate this excess destruction—the less tissue destroyed the quicker healing is achieved. Over-the-counter non-steroidal anti-inflammatory drugs (NSAIDs) include aspirin and ibuprofen; the GP has a wider range of drugs to choose from, including some that are kinder to the stomach.

Pain is treated with analgesics, starting with over-the-counter preparations of paracetamol, ibuprofen or aspirin, followed by paracetamol mixtures on prescription if the pain is not controlled. Strong prescription-only NSAIDs or analgesic drugs may need to be used for acute pain control. Those with a good side-effect profile are to be preferred—the newer COX-2 (cyclooxygenase 2) inhibitors and enantiomeric drugs, like dexketoprofen trometamol, fall into this category (see *Appendix 1, Clinical guidelines for the management of acute low back pain,* pages 51–56). COX-2 inhibitors are probably more appropriate for longer term use. Treating muscle spasm is very effective at reducing pain levels, albeit by a less direct route. Muscle relaxants cited in most texts include diazepam and baclofen; one of the more effective products, methocarbamol, is often overlooked. Early treatment with adequate analgesia with NSAID activity or, NSAID/analgesic combination plus a muscle relaxant is a cocktail that will keep many people mobile and active, the activity being the cornerstone of treatment rather than the medication.

Treatments exclusive to doctors are the various injections used to treat back pain. These range from injections of local anaesthetic, used to identify exactly which structure is causing pain; through epidurals, used to treat disc prolapse by caudal, lumbar or cervical route; to sclerosant injections, for prevention of recurrence in instability conditions. Injections may only be prescribed and administered by doctors trained in these techniques, who may be musculoskeletal physicians, orthopaedic surgeons, rheumatologists or pain specialist anaesthetists.

Some forms of back pain respond very rapidly to an appropriate injection; chronic facet joint strain can be diagnosed when injection of local anaesthetic abolishes the pain immediately. If the pain returns this may be treated successfully by a repeat injection of anaesthetic mixed with a steroid such as triamcinolone. Patients with disc prolapse may avoid surgery by having caudal or lumbar epidural injections or root blocks to ease the pain while the condition regresses naturally. Various mixtures of drugs may be used, including local anaesthetic with or without steroid, small volume steroid or large volume steroid with saline or water.

Discs may be dissolved and removed by chemonucleolysis, in specialist centres, by injection-type treatment.

Of course there is always the possibility of surgery, but only for a very small number of people with back pain.

This may be either as the best option owing to the diagnosis, as in acute spinal stenosis needing decompression, or after all else has failed to alleviate severe intractable pain—when fusion or decompression may help.

*Prevention of recurrence* is achieved by physiotherapy utilizing exercises to build up mobility and strength. Corsets and belts of various types may also be recommended for short periods to allow activity with reduced risk, while strength is being built up by specific exercises. The use of leisure centre gyms by some back pain sufferers is an alternative approach. A recent development in this area is Kieser-Training, which combines medical strengthening training with machines which are computer controlled within a gym environment. This form of training starts by measuring the strength of the back muscles before recommending and monitoring treatment. In this well researched approach there is a direct relationship between pain relief and muscle strengthening in 80% of individuals.

*Homoeopathy* provides a large number of treatments for various aspects of back pain. All homoeopathic treatments work with the natural healing processes. Unlike allopathic treatments, which treat all similar symptoms in different people with the same drug, homoeopathic remedies are chosen by relating the condition to the patient. Therefore different patients with identical symptoms, if such existed, could be given different homoeopathic remedies as their histories and personalities would be different.

Some homoeopathic preparations may be taken generally:

- aconite for fear, anxiety and panic, often associated with back pain
- arnica for injury and bruising, sprains and strains as soon as they happen.

Other remedies linked with back pain have particular associations and include the following:

- *Aesculus hippocastrum:* backs of legs give out; spine feels weak; backache in sacrum and hips, worse on walking or stooping.
- *Cimicifuga racemosa:* spine sensitive: stiffness and contraction in neck and back; lumbar and sacral pain into thighs and hips.
- *Colocynthis:* sciatic pains; stiffness in joints.
- *Gnaphalium:* chronic backache in lumbar region; better resting on back.
- *Guaiacum:* sciatica and lumbago: stinging pain in limbs.
- *Kali carbonicum:* small of back feels weak; burning in spine; lumbago with sudden pains up and down spine to thighs.
- *Nux vomica:* lumbar backache; burning in spine at 3–4 a.m.; sitting is painful; must sit up to turn in bed.
- *Pulsatilla:* shooting pain in nape, back and sacrum after sitting.
- *Rhus toxicodendron:* pain and stiffness in lower back, better with movement or lying on something hard, worse sitting.
- *Valerian:* sciatic pain, worse standing and resting on floor.

As can be seen, the above range of remedies and conditions is wide. The list is included to give some idea of the potential role of homoeopathy in treating acute and chronic back pain. The help of an experienced practitioner is essential to achieve good results.

*Manipulation* is represented by two respected schools which have become regulated by statute in the last few years. Lay practitioners are trained in established colleges, registered and insured, guaranteeing high quality professional treatment. There are slight differences in philosophy, but both recognize the link between structure and function.

Chiropractic was started in 1895 by David D Palmer. Today there are two slightly different training schools: the original chiropractic and McTimoney chiropractic. The basic philosophy considers that almost all conditions producing symptoms may be caused by structural abnormalities in the spine. Diagnosis is by palpation and X-ray examination to identify minute changes in the relative position of adjacent vertebrae. Treatments are performed by small amplitude high speed adjustments focused on the identified malpositions. One characteristic of chiropractic is the moving bed used to help in positioning the patient and during the manipulation. Chiropractic recommends regular maintenance for prevention of a wide range of problems.

Osteopathy was started in 1874 by Andrew T Still. The basic philosophy is that many painful conditions are the result of abnormal function in the joint complexes in the spine. This is the osteopathic lesion of old, now called somatic dysfunction, being 'a dysfunction occurring within the normal range of movement of the joint' causing a variety of symptoms, some associated with the somato-visceral reflex. This explains how some intra-abdominal symptoms are treated by spinal manipulation. Diagnosis follows functional examination and careful joint mobility testing. Treatment is by soft tissue massage, joint positioning and long lever techniques, more recently augmented by various muscle energy techniques.

*Postural therapies* are represented by the Alexander and Feldenkrais techniques, both of which are taught either in groups or one to one. Neither can be learnt from books as both rely on correction of postural anomalies. Teachers can be found through their associations (listed in *Appendix 3*).

*Relaxation* and *hypnosis* are related techniques which have a place in the treatment of back pain—both acute and chronic. Learnt from tapes, books or classes, relaxation works by reducing tension in muscles, thus allowing the bones to realign themselves. The technique requires considerable practice before it can be used to modify pain and muscle spasm.

Self-hypnosis can be useful in controlling acute pain, spasm or anxiety, but in the chronic state may be extremely helpful in boosting confidence to encourage the leap of faith necessary for a sufferer with established chronic pain to start exercising. Hypnosis is an altered state of consciousness developed by the subject with the help or direction of the therapist, and once learnt it can be developed to levels where almost any pain may be tolerated, including minor operations or dental treatment. Therapists may be lay or medically qualified; details of associations are included in *Appendix 3*. Treatment usually follows the onset of pain, but once learnt, the technique will be of use in many circumstances.

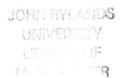

# Rehabilitation

A fairly helpful definition of rehabilitation is 'return to normal living'. However, in general most people survive in a weak physical state. With a lack of general exercise, and an increase in car driving and watching TV from the sofa, back strength and stability is often very poor. This makes it appropriate to describe preventive rehabilitation first, followed by therapeutic rehabilitation for acute and chronic pain.

## Preventive

Preventive exercises are aimed at people with normal lives whose activities—work, domestic, social or sporting—put them at risk of back pain—which is basically everyone. There is a tendency for muscles to weaken over time (Figure 8); however, the body has tolerances which have to be used up before symptoms occur. Without objective testing no one knows how close they are to getting symptoms.

The aims of preventive exercise are increased flexibility, strength and stability. Strength is important in the abdominal muscles, especially the oblique and transversus muscles, posterior paraspinal muscles and quadratus lumborum.

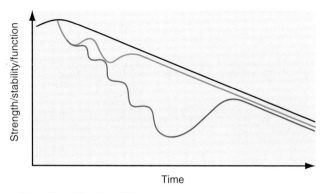

— Normal loss of function with time
— Acute episodes adequately treated
— Failure of adequate treatment with resultant chronic back pain
— Chronic pain management and rehab still possible

**Figure 8**
*Natural decay of function compared with that in acute and chronic pain.*

## Exercises

*Sit-ups* should be performed with knees bent and toes free, reaching forward with the hands either side of the thighs. It is only necessary to lift the shoulder blades from the floor, not to move to a sitting position. This basic exercise may be modified by increasing the number of repetitions and repeat sets, and may be graduated by moving the arms to cross the chest, then held above the head. Recruitment of the transversus muscle by pulling in the tummy button before each sit-up and use of the oblique muscle by rotating the elbow alternately to the opposite knee further aids the effectiveness of this exercise, especially if done slowly. The role of the abdominal muscles is shown in Figure 9.

*Side bending*. Standing and bending to either side with weights in each hand strengthens the lateral muscles.

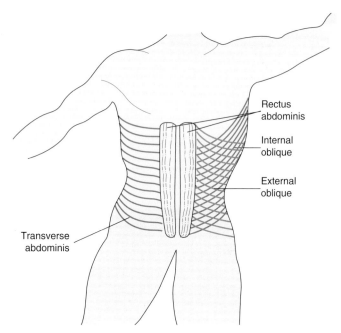

**Figure 9**
*The combined effect of the abdominal muscles in structuring the abdominal wall is the production of a waist and a firm tubular structure which supports the spine.*

*Back extension.* This is done by lying on the floor face down with hands behind the back, then lifting the head and shoulders up as far as possible. Again this may be augmented by increasing the number of repetititions, moving the hands to behind the head, lifting the legs as well and rotating alternately to either side.

Once these exercises have been mastered, all the exercises available in a gym or exercise manual may be added.

*Stretching* to increase flexibility is necessary to establish a balance in the muscles. This is especially true with regard

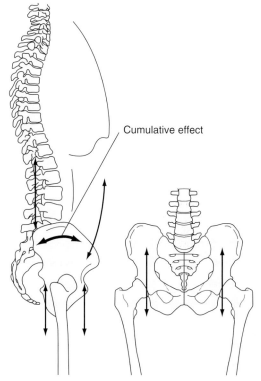

**Figure 10**
*Pelvic tilt. Muscles working about the sacroiliac and hip joints must be balanced above and below, front and back, and side to side.*

to hamstrings, quadriceps, abdominal and lower back muscles working round the pelvis. Muscles may only be balanced by stretching.

- Hamstring muscles in the back of the thigh are stretched by putting the foot on a chair and leaning forward with the knee straight until a stretching is felt. As progress is made the height of the foot can be raised. Each leg should be worked on separately until they are equal.

- Quadriceps femoris muscles at the front of the thigh are stretched by pulling the heel up to the buttock, holding just above the ankle.
- By sitting on the floor and reaching forward the lower back is stretched and the spine is flexed.
- The abdominal muscles are stretched and the spine is extended by doing a press-up from a prone position with the pelvis remaining in contact with the floor.

Coordination training with a wobble-board, Swiss ball or similar apparatus to coordinate muscle function is the final element of full preparation for even normal everyday activity. If any form of physical exercise is undertaken, specific muscle strengthening, mobility training, coordination and skills training will need to be planned. This is basic risk prevention—like looking both ways before you cross the road.

Heart–lung and stamina training, although not obviously linked to back health, increase the ability to cope with stress. Stress is often manifested in muscular tension in back, neck and shoulder muscles, offering a link with some back complaints.

## *Following acute pain episodes*

Rehabilitation starts as soon after the onset of pain as possible. Areas not affected by the pain should continue to be used normally. As soon as the pain is controlled and the sufferer reassured that no major injury or disease process is involved, local movement is encouraged within the normal range, up to the onset of pain in every direction. This begins the process of maintaining flexibility; once the flexibility approaches normal, strengthening should start. Symmetry is important with the flexibility. Strengthening needs to be planned sequentially: to correct pre-existing weakness, to treat weakness secondary to the problem and to add strength for prevention. The help of an experienced physio-therapist or fitness instructor may make this process quicker and more effective. A second pair of eyes with a knowledge of the muscles may prevent aggravation of the problem whilst focusing training on appropriate groups of muscles.

From the point where pain is removed and function acceptable it is imperative that further exercise as outlined above is undertaken to reduce the risk of recurrence and chronicity.

## *Following chronic or recurrent episodes*

Chronic pain or frequent recurrences do not indicate more severe problems, they just reflect the failure to treat the earlier episodes adequately. The difference is that the number of restricted movements or weak muscles will be greater, together with a more disrupted coordination system. The hill to climb will be longer, not necessarily steeper (Figure 11).

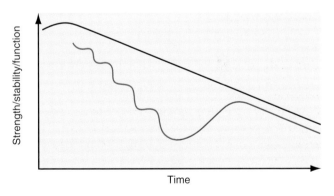

— Normal loss of function with time
— Failure of adequate treatment with resultant chronic back pain
— Chronic pain management and rehab still possible

**Figure 11**
*Function in chronic back pain compared with normal natural decay of function.*

Rehabilitation at this stage must go hand in hand with psychological support and full reassurance that major conditions are not involved in the pain process. This requires a very comprehensive examination, possibly with further investigation, blood samples, X-ray examination or magnetic resonance imaging (MRI) scan, if indicated, to gain a full explanation of the likely pain generation process. The first part of the hill at this stage is convincing the sufferer to start an exercise programme when they are in pain. The programme planned must be gradual, progressive and non-threatening, allowing the sufferer to dictate the pace, which will gradually build up as confidence returns.

As progress continues the types of exercise are extended, based around those for prevention outlined above, but with fewer repeats to start with and only gradual progression.

With exercises of any kind related to back pain, sufferers cannot do too few repeats to start with, but it is common to do too many. Start with two or three exercises done properly only two or three times and build up to five or more before doing two or three sets of repeats, e.g. six sit-ups repeated two or three times with a short break between sets.

**Treatment of established chronic pain**

Although not really the remit of this book, it is necessary to hold hope for those for whom it seems too late. There are well recognised treatment programmes for those with established chronic back pain. These can be broken down into four areas in parallel with other parts of the book.

- Treating pain by changing analgesics from the current medications to another group and by adding in pain-modifying drugs such as amitriptyline or carbamazepine.

- Psychological support with either counselling, group activities, self-support groups and reassurance of the absence of a disease process, or with antidepressants.
- Homoeopathic remedies may be used for either of the above two indications (see *Treatment*).
- Monitored, focused and graduated exercises with stretching strengthening and balancing of muscle groups using Kieser-Training, Pilates, tai-chi or yoga-type programmes. Stamina training using rhythmic exercises and improving general heart and lung fitness.

## Acute pain, chronic pain and the transition between them

Pain is defined as: a sensory and emotional experience associated with actual or potential tissue damage or described in such terms.

The sensory aspect ranges from mild discomfort to agonizing pain (1–100 on the visual analogue scale). The emotional aspect, which is often overlooked and blamed as an over-reaction, ranges from apprehension to abject panic. Most doctors concentrate on the sensory pain and its complex causes rather than the simple treatment. Sometimes the emotional panic may be easier to treat with explanation and reassurance, in the first instance.

## Types of pain

Various types of pain have been defined.

*Acute physiological pain,* as discussed earlier, is the direct result of stimulation of nociceptors, whether mechanically, thermally or chemically, and is an important protective mechanism, warning of intense or noxious stimuli. By direct connections from the dorsal to the ventral horns of the spinal cord, the withdrawal reflex is activated (see

Figure 12). Sustained physiological pain leads to sustained withdrawal reflex. Flexor muscle spasm occurs with the generation of further tenderness in the tensed muscles.

*Clinical pain* has three features as defined by Woolf (1994), the pain is spontaneous, pain responses to noxious stimuli are exaggerated and pain is produced by normal stimuli like pressure, heat or movement. This spectrum of hypersensitivity, hyperalgesia and allodynia affects two zones, the zone of primary hyperalgesia, e.g. the site of a bruise in an area of tissue damage, and the zone of secondary hyperalgesia, in surrounding tissue which is undamaged. Primary hyperalgesia is caused by a phenomenon called peripheral sensitization resulting from the release of inflammatory mediators by damaged tissues, which is well researched and documented. However, this is not the whole story, as the area of hyperalgesia is wider than the spread of these media-tors. Peripheral sensitization does not fully explain all the features of clinical pain, especially the pain response to normal joint movement (mechanical hypersensitivity) as in arthritic joints.

This sensation represents a misinterpretation of normal sensory inputs as pain, described recently as central sensitization. This represents a change in the function of neurons in the dorsal horn of the spinal cord, referred to as neuronal plasticity. Central sensitization is induced by peripheral nociceptor stimuli arriving in the dorsal horn cells via unmyelinated C fibres (Figure 12). In this area they cause the release of at least two neurotransmitters which alter mechanoreceptor and thermal receptor neurons post-synaptically to become sensitive and induce a pain sensation instead of their original message (neuronal plasticity). The area covered by these neurons is much larger than the area of original injury, hence, secondary hyperalgesia and allodynia. Once started, central sensitization persists for a relatively long time,

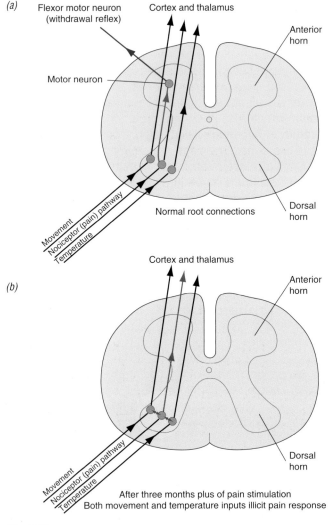

**Figure 12**
*Simplified central sensitization. (a) The pathways for movement, pain and temperature are normally separate. (b) However, after several months of pain stimulation, although the pain pathway may no longer be receiving pain stimulation because the source of pain has healed, both the movement and temperature sensors are inputting 'illicit' pain responses because of a 'short circuit' between nerve cells.*

even after the triggering cause has healed or disappeared.

In back pain, with strong psychological implications, these phenomena are of particular interest and paramount importance. Statements such as 'if I have pain like this there must be a cause', 'I've had the pain for ages so the cause must be getting worse', regularly confront doctors. These very reasonable fears require significant reassurance. Sprains and strains can reasonably be expected to heal in a maximum of 6 weeks, like any cut which can be seen on the skin. Injuries in the back cannot be seen to heal; recurrent episodes, encouraged by failure to rehabilitate, lead to central sensitization, then movement itself causes pain. Not surprisingly, the end result is panic.

Experimental pharmacology suggests that mechanical hyperalgesia requires the coactivation of two receptors on neurons in the spinal cord, primarily mediated by cyclooxygenase products of arachidonic acid metabolism.

> Woolf and Chong (1993) suggested that in view of the discovery of central sensitization 'it is clinically more useful to prevent central sensitization than attempt to treat it once established'. In terms of a practical approach to back pain, this means adequate sustained analgesia as soon as possible after the onset of the stimulus.

Which sounds like a good reason to use NSAIDs in the early treatment of acute back pain.

Discussions of the time period relating to the transition from acute physiological pain to chronic clinical pain are inconclusive, but depend somewhat on the psychological state of the sufferer at the onset and the intensity of the pain initially rather more than on other factors. Time frames of between 6 and 12 weeks for the establishment of the chronic state fit reasonably well with the International Association for the Study of Pain (IASP) definition of chronic pain as being 'present for or recurrent over a period of 3–6 months', for the standardization of trial protocols.

For doctors and patients alike this means a very narrow window of approximately 3 months to effectively treat acute back pain and to prevent chronicity. As a large proportion of back pain settles in 6 weeks, but may go on to be recurrent, a pragmatic view would be to treat back pain that is persistent for 3 weeks or more vigorously by all means possible. The window becomes 3 weeks to avoid recurrence and 9 weeks to avoid the establishment of a chronic state. This accords well with the Royal College of General Practitioners guidelines, but is at odds with the availability of treatment—the typical waiting time for physiotherapy being 6 weeks, 4–6 months being the norm for a hospital consultant appointment.

# Examination

The art of clinical examination has been overtaken by the drive for 'validated data collection', on patients: when a new patient is seen and asked to remove clothing so that the spine can be examined, getting down to skin requires constant encouragement. A great deal of information can be garnered by looking at the patient during this 'unaccustomed' manoeuvre. Balance, general joint mobility and the adoption of trick movements to avoid certain positions are all useful pointers, even before the examination proper begins. A warm room with space to watch walking gait helps, but time to conduct the examination is the most valuable tool. General spinal examination will be described below; more detailed texts are included in *Appendix 2*.

## Static observation

View the posture from the back and side, noting head position, shoulder height, scoliosis (thoracic or lumbar), deviation, balance, waist skin creases, leg length, pronation of the foot and pes planus.

## Global movements

Ask the patient to move as directed as far as possible without suffering pain. This reassures them and encourages them to show what they can do. Provided that no pain is experienced, increased effort to move may be encouraged to give the best range of movement. Observation of movement range, symmetry and spine shape is required.

---

- Flexion is measured either by reaching down the leg, distance to the floor, finger tips, knuckles or palms on the floor.
- Extension is measured using hands behind the thighs and knee crease for rough assessment of movement.
- Side bending is measured by reference to the fingertip–knee crease distance.

---

## Dural signs

Watching the patient ascend the couch to take up a supine position is very illuminating; if they can sit with legs outstretched this equates with full straight leg raising (SLR), suspicious if subsequently SLR testing is less than 90°. 'Genuine' patients may move very carefully and slowly, but will almost always apologize for doing so, unlike the malingerer, who often exhibits jerky movements and exaggerated responses. Professor Gordon Waddell has published extensively on non-organic signs, which makes useful reading.

According to Cyriax, central disc protrusion with dural irritation gives bilateral SLR limitation with pain, whereas lateral protrusion gives unilateral limitation of SLR and pain in the distribution of the relevant nerve—L4, L5, S1 or S2. Paraesthesia, numbness and weakness in the root distribution with reflex changes indicates a degree of pressure on the nerve, rather than dural irritation. Muscle strength testing and reflexes in the limb give a strong indication of the level of any root compression (see Figures 5 and 6 and Table 2).

## *Specific spine examination*

Relative muscle tightness/balance about the pelvis should be tested by SLR for hamstrings, knee flexion for quadriceps, and hip extension for psoas (see Figure 10). The sacroiliac joint is stressed and palpated for tenderness, symptoms from this joint giving low back pain which may refer through to the groin.

Spasm seen or felt in the paraspinal muscles, tenderness reported by the patient on palpation of the muscles and facet joints, found two finger breadths from the spine processes, helps to identify a level which may correspond with the symptoms. Detailed segmental assessment of mobility needs apprenticeship-style teaching, as provided at the London College of Osteopathic Medicine.

This brief examination routine will augment the identification of red flag conditions which all doctors will recognize, allowing subsequent reassurance of the sufferer to be more robust. With a little practice, the identification of patients who would benefit from some form of more vigorous intervention (manipulation, injection therapy or strengthening) would ensue. Satisfaction in treating back pain patients could follow, instead of panic on the part of the practitioner.

## Chronic spinal stenosis

Pressure is the cause of pain in chronic spinal stenosis, but by a different mechanism to that described earlier. Multiple lesions into the spinal canal, osteophytes, disc bulges or other obstructions cause raised venous pressure. With activity, such as walking, the blood flow increases but the venous flow reaches a limit imposed by the obstructions, causing back pressure which reduces the arterial circulation to the spinal canal. Rising pressure and reducing circulation results in ischaemia, producing diffuse buttock, leg or calf pain which comes on with exercise and is relieved by rest or leaning forward. This latter alleviating factor causes confusion, as patients can walk further and faster uphill than downhill, because walking downhill causes extension of the spine and closure of the spinal canal. This is in contrast to an acute occurrence requiring emergency surgical correction following a central disc prolapse at the L4–5 level into a small spinal canal where the sacral nerve roots are compressed, giving buttock pain, leg pain, paraesthesia and saddle anaesthesia together with sphincter distur-bances.

# Fibromyalgia syndrome

This extremely interesting condition tells us a significant amount about the relationship between the musculoskeletal system and sleep. Fibromyalgia syndrome (FMS) is a chronic non-degenerative, non-progressive, non-inflammatory, truly systemic pain condition. Diseases have known causes and well understood mechanisms for producing symptoms. FMS is a syndrome, which means it is a specific set of signs and symptoms that occur together. It is characterized by tender points in muscles from the base of the skull to the lower thoracic region and from the neck down the arms, and is associated with poor sleep patterns. The official research definition requires that tender points must be present in all four quadrants of the body—i.e. the upper right and left and lower right and left parts of the body. There must be widespread, more-or-less continuous pain for at least 3 months. Tender points can fluctuate and vary from day to day and even from hour to hour. Tender points occur in pairs on various parts of the body; as such, the pain is usually distributed equally on both sides of the body. In FMS, tender points are present at 18 'official' points.

Sleep, or the lack of it, plays a crucial role in FMS, i.e. not getting enough sleep, or the right kind of sleep in particular. People with FMS often have the alpha–delta sleep anomaly. As soon as deep delta level sleep is reached, alpha waves intrude and cause awakening or change to a lighter stage of sleep. Waking feeling traumatized is the sign of unrestorative sleep. The body heals and our neurotransmitters and other informational substances are restored and regulated during delta sleep. This condition responds best to amitriptyline at low doses to restore normal sleep patterns, with resolution of the tender points.

## Non-back pain

A variety of conditions occurring in internal organs may lead to back pain. Few would argue that referral from kidney stone or infection, penetrating posterior duodenal ulcer, gall bladder disease, pleural inflammation, subphrenic abscess or gynaecological conditions may present with back pain from upper thoracic to lower lumbar levels. These conditions may be affected by spinal movements and produce tenderness in the tissues of the back on examination, causing difficulty with diagnosis. The opposite is also true; right loin pain with normal kidney and gall bladder investigations may result from spinal dysfunction. Identification of this possibility before exploratory operation may save the patient from undergoing hazardous procedures and save the health service much-needed funds.

The February 1999 edition of these guidelines is reproduced on the following pages with the permission of the Royal College of General Practitioners.

Further information and copies of the full evidence base for these guidelines are available from:
Paula-Jayne McDowell
Royal College of General Practitioners
14 Princes Gate
Hyde Park
London SW7 1PU.
http://www.rcgp.org.uk

*Contributing organizations:
Royal College of General Practitioners
Chartered Society of Physiotherapy
British Osteopathic Association
British Chiropractic Association
National Back Pain Association (now BackCare)

Review date: December 2001.

These brief clinical guidelines and their supporting base of research evidence are intended to assist in the management of acute low back pain. They present a synthesis of up-to-date international evidence and make recommendations on case management. Recommendations and evidence relate primarily to the first 6 weeks of an episode, when management decisions may be required in a changing clinical picture. However, the guidelines may also be useful in the sub-acute period.

These guidelines have been constructed by a multi-professional group and subjected to extensive professional review. They are intended to be used as a guide by the whole range of health professionals who advise people with acute low back pain, particularly simple backache, in the NHS and in private practice.

*Psychosocial 'yellow flags'*
When conducting assessment, it may be useful to consider psychosocial 'yellow flags' (beliefs or behaviours on the part of the patient which may predict poor outcomes).

The following factors are important and consistently predict poor outcomes:

- a belief that back pain is harmful or potentially severely disabling
- fear-avoidance behaviour and reduced activity levels
- tendency to low mood and withdrawal from social interaction
- expectation of passive treatment(s) rather than a belief that active participation will help.

# Diagnostic triage

Diagnostic triage is the differential diagnosis between:
* Simple backache (non-specific low back pain)
* Nerve root pain
* Possible serious spinal pathology

**Simple backache:** *specialist referral not required*
* Presentation 20–55 years
* Lumbosacral, buttocks and thighs
* 'Mechanical' pain
* Patient well

**Nerve root pain:** *specialist referral not generally required within first 4 weeks, provided resolving*
* Unilateral leg pain worse than low back pain
* Radiates to foot or toes
* Numbness and paraesthesia in same distribution
* SLR reproduces leg pain
* Localized neurological signs

**Red flags for *possible* serious spinal pathology**: *consider prompt investigation or referral (less than 4 weeks)*
* Presentation under age 20 or onset over 55
* Non-mechanical pain
* Thoracic pain
* Past history – carcinoma, steroids, HIV
* Unwell, weight loss
* Widespread neurological symptoms or signs
* Structural deformity

**Cauda equina syndrome:** *emergency referral*
* Sphincter disturbance
* Gait disturbance
* Saddle anaesthesia

---

**On the next two pages the evidence is weighted as follows:**
*** Generally consistent finding in a majority of acceptable studies.
** Either based on a single acceptable study, or a weak or inconsistent finding in some of multiple acceptable studies.
* Limited scientific evidence, which does not meet all the criteria of 'acceptable' studies.

---

# *Principal recommendations*

## *Assessment*
- Carry out diagnostic triage (see previous page)
- X-rays are not routinely indicated in simple backache
- Consider psychosocial 'yellow flags' (see page 52)

---

## Simple backache

### *Drug therapy*
- Prescribe analgesics at regular intervals, not p.r.n.
- Start with paracetamol. If inadequate, substitute NSAIDs (e.g. ibuprofen or diclofenac) and then paracetamol-weak opioid compound (e.g. codydramol or coproxamol). Finally, consider adding a short course of muscle relaxant (e.g. diazepam or baclofen)
- Avoid strong opioids if possible

### *Bed rest*
- Do not recommend or use bed rest as a treatment
- Some patients may be confined to bed for a few days as a consequence of their pain but this should not be considered a treatment

### *Advice on staying active*
- Advise patients to stay as active as possible and to continue normal daily activities
- Advise patients to increase their physical activities progressively over a few days or weeks
- If a patient is working, then advice to stay at work or return to work as soon as possible is probably beneficial

### *Manipulation*
- Consider manipulative treatment for patients who need additional help with pain relief or who are failing to return to normal daily activities

### *Back exercises*
- Referral for reactivation/rehabilitation should be considered for patients who have not returned to ordinary activities and work by 6 weeks

# *Evidence*

* Diagnostic triage forms the basis for referral, investigation and management
* Royal College of Radiologists Guidelines
*** Psychosocial factors play an important role in low back pain and disability and influence the patient's response to treatment and rehabilitation

---

** Paracetamol effectively reduces low back pain
*** NSAIDs effectively reduce pain. Ibuprofen and diclofenac have lower risks of GI complications
** Paracetamol-weak opioid compounds may be effective when NSAIDs or paracetamol alone are inadequate
*** Muscle relaxants effectively reduce low back pain

*** Bed rest for 2–7 days is worse than placebo or ordinary activity and is not as effective as alternative treatments for relief of pain, rate of recovery, return to daily activities and work

*** Advice to continue ordinary activity can give equivalent or faster symptomatic recovery from the acute attack and lead to less chronic disability and less time off work

*** Manipulation can provide short-term improvement in pain and activity levels and higher patient satisfaction
** The optimum timing for this intervention is unclear
** The risks of manipulation are very low in skilled hands

*** It is doubtful that specific back exercises produce clinically significant improvement in acute low back pain
** There is some evidence that exercise programmes and physical reconditioning can improve pain and functional levels in patients with chronic low back pain. There are theoretical arguments for starting this at around 6 weeks

# Key patient information points

## Simple backache
*– give positive message*

- There is nothing to worry about. Backache is very common.
- No sign of any serious damage or disease. Full recovery in days or weeks – but may vary.
- No permanent weakness. Recurrence possible – but does not mean reinjury.
- Activity is helpful, too much rest is not. Hurting does not mean harm.

## Nerve root pain
*– give guarded positive messages*

- No cause for alarm. No sign of disease.
- Conservative treatment should suffice – but may take a month or two.
- Full recovery expected – but recurrence possible.

## Possible serious spinal pathology
*– avoid negative messages*

- Some tests are needed to make the diagnosis.
- Often these tests are negative.
- The specialist will advise on the best treatment.
- Rest or activity avoidance until appointment to see specialist.

## Patient booklet

The above messages can be enhanced by an educational booklet given at consultation. *The Back Book* is an evidence-based booklet developed for use with these guidelines, and is published by The Stationery Office, London (ISBN 011 702 0788).

# Appendix 2
# References and further reading

Baldry PE, *Trigger Points and Musculoskeletal Pain*, 2nd edn. Edinburgh: Churchill Livingstone, 1996.

Brune K, Spinal cord effects of antipyretic analgesics. *Drugs* 1994; **47** (Suppl 5): 21–27.

Croft PR, Macfarlane J, Papageorgiou C et al, Outcome of low back pain in general practice: a prospective study. *Br Med J* 1998; **316**: 1356–59.

Cyriax JA, *Textbook of Orthopaedic Medicine,* 11th edn. London: Baillière Tindall, 1984.

Cyriax JH, Cyriax PJ, *Cyriax's Illustrated Manual of Orthopaedic Medicine,* 2nd edn. Oxford: Butterworh-Heinemann, 1996.

Dorman T, Ravin T, *Diagnosis and Injection Techniques in Orthopaedic Medicine.* Baltimore, MD: Williams & Wilkins, 1991.

Dvorak J, Dvorak V, *Manual Medicine – Diagnostics,* 2nd edn. Stuttgart: Thieme, 1990.

Gill KP, Callaghan MJ, The measurement of lumbar proproception in individuals with and without low back pain. *Spine* 1998; **23**: 371–77.

Gunn CC, *The Gunn Approach to the Treatment of Chronic Pain*, 2nd edn. Edinburgh: Churchill Livingstone, 1996.

Hackett GS, *Ligament and Tendon Relaxation Treated by Prolotherapy*, 3rd edn. Springfield, IL: Charles C Thomas, 1958.

Hartman L, *Handbook of Osteopathic Technique,* 3rd edn. Cheltenham: Stanely Thornes, 1996.

Hutson MA, *Back Pain Recognition and Management.* Oxford: Butter-worth-Heinemann, 1993.

Jayson MIV, *Lumbar Spine and Back Pain,* 4th edn. Edinburgh: Churchill Livingstone, 1992.

Lewit K, *Manipulative Therapy of the Locomotor System,* 3rd edn. Oxford: Butterworth-Heinemann, 1997.

Lewit K, Chain reactions in the locomotor system in the light of co-activation patterns based on the developmental neurology. *J Orth Med* 1999; **21**: 52–7.

Maigne R, *Diagnosis and Treatment of Pain of Vertebral Origin: A Manual Medicine Approach.* Baltimore: Lippincott, Williams and Wilkins, 1996.

Mann F, *Acupuncture: Cure of Many Diseases,* 2nd edn. Oxford: Butterworth-Heinemann, 1992.

McCormack KJ, The spinal actions of nonsteroidal anti-inflammatory drugs and the dissociation between their anti-inflammatory and analgesic effects. *Drugs* 1994; **47** (Suppl 5): 28–45.

Meller ST, Gebhart GF, Spinal mediators of hyperalgesia. *Drugs* 1994; **47** (Suppl 5): 10–20.

Mottram S, Comerford M, Stability dysfunction and low back pain. *J Orth Med* 1998; **20**: 13–18.

Rosen M [Chair], *Back Pain: Report of CSAG Committee on Back Pain*, 4th impression 1996, The Stationary Office Books, 1994, UK – association with Department of Health.

Sambrook PN, MacGregor AJ, Spector TD, Genetic influences on cervical and lumbar disc degeneration: A magnetic resonance imaging study in twins. *Arthritis Rheum* 1999; **42**: 366–72.

Tanner J, BHMA, *Beating Back Pain: A Practical Self-help Guide to Prevention and Treatment.* London: Dorling Kindersley, 1991.

Travell JG, Simons DG, *Myofascial Pain and Dysfunction: The Trigger Point Manual: The Lower Extremities* – Vol 2. Baltimore: Williams and Wilkins, 1992.

Volinn E, The epidemiology of back pain in the rest of the world. *Spine* 1997; **22**: 1747.

Vroomen PCAJ et al, Lack of effectiveness of bed rest for sciatica. *N Engl J Med* 1999; **340**: 418–23.

Waddell G, McCulloch JA, Kummel E, Venner RM, Nonorganic physical signs in low-back pain. *Spine* 1980; **5**: 117–25.

Waddell G, *The Back Pain Revolution.* Edinburgh: Churchill Livingstone, 1998.

Wall PD, Melzak R, *Challenge of Pain,* 2nd edn. Harmondsworth: Penguin Science, 1996.

Woolf CJ, A new strategy for the treatment of inflammatory pain: Prevention or elimination of central sensitization. *Drugs* 1994; **47** (Suppl 5): 1–9.

Woolf CJ, Chong M-S, Preemptive analgesia: treating postoperative pain by preventing the establishment of central sensitization. *Anesth Analg* 1993; **77**: 1–18.

**BackCare**
14 Elm Tree Avenue
Teddington TW11 8ST
*Tel:* 020 8977 5474

**British Chiropractic Association**
Blagrave House
Blagrave Street
Reading RG1 1QB
*Tel:* 0118 950 5950

**British Institute of Musculoskeletal Medicine**
34 Park Avenue
Watford WD1 3NS
*Tel:* 01923 220 999

**British Medical Acupuncture Society**
Royal London Homoeopathic Hospital
60 Great Ormond Street
London WC1N 3HR
*Tel:* 020 7278 1615

**British School of Osteopathy**
1–4 Suffolk Street
London SW1Y 4HG
*Tel:* 020 7407 0222

**British Society of Experimental and Clinical Hypnosis**
*Hon Sec:* Mrs Phyllis Alden
c/o Department of Clinical Oncology
Derbyshire Royal Infirmary
London Road
Derby DE1 2QY
*Tel:* 01332 347 141, Extn: 4150

**British Society of Medical and Dental Hypnosis**
23 Broadfields Heights
53/58 Broadfields Avenue
Edgware HA8 8PF
*Tel:* 020 8905 4342 or 020 8958 8069

**The Feldenkrais Guild UK**
PO Box 370
London N10 3XA
*For information contact:*
Leila Malcolm
East Holcombe
Shillingford
Tiverton
Devon EX16 9BR
*Tel:* 019398 361 300
*email:* 106222.1342@compuserve.com

**Kieser-Training**
Greater London House
Hampstead Road
London NW1 7DF
*Tel:* 020 7391 9980 or 020 7391 9988

**London College of Osteopathic Medicine**
8–10 Boston Place
London NW1 6QH
*Tel:* 020 7262 5250

**McTimoney Chiropractic College**
The Clock House
22–26 Ock Street
Abingdon
Oxon OX14 5NY
*Tel:* 01235 523336
*email:* chiropractice@mctimoney-college.ac.uk

**Society of Teachers of the Alexander Technique**
20 London House
266 Fulham Road
London SW10 9EL
*Tel:* 020 7351 0828

# Index

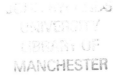